N

PLAB

PART 1 EMQ

POCKET BOOK 2

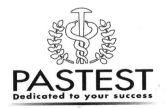

PLAB

PART 1 EMQ

POCKET BOOK 2

Peter Kroker

MB BS, BA, MRCP
Consultant Physician and Geriatrician
Department for Medicine of Ageing,
Chelsea and Westminster Hospital, London

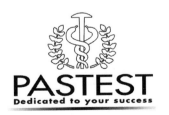

PASTEST
Dedicated to your success

© 2001 PASTEST LTD
Egerton Court, Parkgate Estate,
Knutsford, Cheshire, WA16 8DX
Telephone: 01565 752000

First edition 2001
Reprinted 2001, 2002, 2003

A catalogue record for this book is available from the British Library.

ISBN: 1 901198 62 6

The information contained within this book was obtained by the author from reliable sources. However, while every effort has been made to ensure its accuracy, no responsibility for loss, damage or injury occasioned to any person acting or refraining from action as a result of information contained herein can be accepted by the publishers or authors.

Typeset by Breeze Limited, Manchester
Printed by Athenaeum Press Ltd, Tyne and Wear

CONTENTS

INTRODUCTION

About this book

Congratulations on buying this book!

Unfortunately, not everyone can pass PLAB Part 1 first time. At the time of writing, there are only a few books on the market that are designed to help you revise for the exam. Amazingly, many candidates do not buy any books or go on any courses. Whilst using this book, or any book, cannot guarantee a pass at the next exam, it will certainly improve your chances.

The proportion of candidates that pass is fixed at each sitting. Therefore, you are in competition with everyone that sits the exam at the same time as you. If you help one of your friends with their revision, you may be helping them pass instead of you. Group learning is, of course, often of great benefit, but be careful that you are not helping others more than yourself. For your own sake, do not lend this book to anyone else until you have passed the exam…

This book is not a textbook. You will not find great detail and many topics could not be included in the space available. A small textbook or guide (such as the Oxford Handbook series) is recommended for revision. Subjects like paediatrics, obstetrics and psychiatry seem popular with the examiners. If you are weak in these areas, it might be worth obtaining small books dedicated to these specialities. Do not spend too much time or money on new, large textbooks. You will never read them.

This book is not, strictly speaking, a revision book. There are very few lists in the text. Again, this is partly due to the limited number of topics that could be covered. Also, there are some very good books of lists and differential diagnosis already in print. If you like lists and your memory can cope with them, then it may be worth buying one of these books.

If you are new to the exam, this book will introduce you to the type of question that you will be facing. For those of you who have already sat the new exam (since July 2000), the book provides another 200 practice questions. Many difficult questions are made easier by understanding the way in which an examiner might think. I hope to provide some insight into the way in which the questions and answers are designed. This is particularly important now that the General Medical Council (GMC) has changed the format of the exam.

The new exam and why it was changed

The General Medical Council (GMC) frequently reviews the way in which it examines overseas doctors in the PLAB process. Ultimately the exam may be replaced by another form of assessment. In the meantime, the GMC is keen to make the exam fairer and open to independent scrutiny. The previous Part 1 (multiple choice, picture and clinical problem-solving questions) was not felt to be a fair test of knowledge and ability.

A number of books were available for the previous model of exam. If you have any of these books, do not throw them away. The topics that are covered are still those that the PLAB exam will test. Incidentally, there is no guarantee that the exam format will not change again in the future.

Multiple choice questions (MCQs) are particularly subject to criticism. The new exam consists of Extended Matching Questions (EMQs), closely modelled on the style of exams in the USA. According to the GMC, the level of knowledge required to pass the new exam should be roughly the same as before. At the first sitting of the new exam, it was felt to be harder than expected by many candidates.

The GMC states that the standard required is that of a first year Senior House Officer, i.e. someone with 12 to 18 months experience since qualification. Some questions in July 2000 were almost certainly harder than that and seemed to expect greater depth of knowledge. Do not let this discourage you. A hard exam is equally hard on everyone. An easy exam is more likely to let weaker candidates pass by luck alone.

Many candidates do not always answer all 200 questions, you will need to practice using the time wisely. There will always be a few questions that you struggle with, try to waste as little time as possible on these. Put down an educated guess and move on quickly to a question you feel more confident about. This will boost your morale and produce greater time efficiency.

Since July 2000 there have been no picture questions in the Part 1 exam. The GMC would not commit to whether picture questions will be reintroduced in the future.

Are EMQs harder than MCQs?

This is a difficult question to answer. MCQs are easy to set and mark. They test recall (often short term memory) and do not attempt to simulate clinical reality. A guess at multiple choice gives you a 50/50 chance of a correct answer. So does tossing a coin. An educated guess is often not much better due to the nature of the question. You either know it, or you don't.

EMQs are much harder to write. They test knowledge and deduction and often attempt to simulate clinical problem-solving. A random guess is unlikely to produce a correct answer when there may be as many as 14 possibilities. An educated guess is more likely to be right than wrong.

EMQs are probably a better test of knowledge and experience than MCQs. In clinical practice, if a 25-year-old man attends casualty with left-sided chest pain you do not think like this:

'Sudden unilateral chest pain in a 25-year-old man is commonly due to
*   pulmonary embolism – True*
*   pneumothorax – True*
*   dissecting thoracic aortic aneurysm – False'*

Whereas you might think the following:

'The most likely cause of sudden left-sided chest pain in a 25-year-old
man is a pneumothorax'

EMQs also test the application of knowledge. In the July 2000 exam, most of the questions asked candidates to select the best investigation, rather than the most likely diagnosis. This is also relevant to clinical practice and harder to answer. When faced with the patient with chest pain, you will have a differential diagnosis and need to plan investigations to decide which diagnosis is correct. You may think the differential diagnosis is between pneumothorax, pulmonary embolism and oesophagitis. You must then decide whether a chest X-ray, arterial blood gases or an endoscopy is the investigation of choice. There may not be one single investigation that will establish the diagnosis in all circumstances, so you must pick the most discriminatory one. In this instance, a chest X-ray is probably the most useful test.

In answer to the question 'are EMQs harder than MCQs?', the answer is probably 'Yes'. However, they are a better and fairer test of clinical ability.

Doctors who pass this new exam will be those who have combined reading with hands-on experience. The previous Part 1 exam could, potentially, be passed by someone who had never seen a patient.

How to use this book

This book is designed as a complete mock PLAB Part 1 Examination. In the front section of this book there are 200 EMQs covering a wide selection of topics. The second section has answers to the questions with detailed, but not exhaustive, explanations to the answers. In the appendix, you will find a table of normal values for standard laboratory tests and a list of some drugs whose names or spellings are different in the UK to other countries.

Endeavour to use the practice exam **under strict examination conditions**: make sure you set aside a full three hours for the exam, preferably during the daytime when the real exam will take place. Make sure you are not disturbed in any way – unplug the telephone, do not have any background music on and make sure your partner or flatmate is out of the way.

Work systematically through the exam paper from the beginning. Previous candidates found that some questions were considerably harder than others. If a question is obviously difficult, miss it out and move on to the next one. If the whole topic is unfamiliar to you, move on to the next one. Two minutes are more efficiently spent answering two easy questions than puzzling over one hard question. When you reach the end of the paper, go back to the questions you missed out until you run out of time. Three hours is not a long time to answer 200 questions, you have slightly less than one minute per question.

When the three hours have finished, stop answering questions. Relax and treat yourself, you deserve it!

When you are refreshed, come back and finish any questions you did not answer during the time on a separate sheet of paper. If you completed all 200 questions, well done! If not, have a go at all the others – an educated guess is often the right answer. Then go through the answers and mark the questions you managed during the time and see how you did. Look at the other questions separately. Use the explanations to identify areas of strength and weakness to guide your revision. It is difficult to say what score you will need to pass the exam, as the pass mark will vary at each sitting, depending on the difficulty of the exam. I would expect that a score of at least 50–60% would be a bare minimum to pass. In January 2001, the pass rate was 60%.

It is unlikely that you will remember many of the questions in this book for long. About a week before the real thing, it will be worth trying this practice exam again. In using this book, you are making sure that the exam is not the first time you have encountered this type of question. Hopefully, the next PLAB Part 1 Exam will be the last one you have to take.

Referring to our Revision Checklist at the back of this book will ensure that you cover the most popular examination themes. We have also included a comprehensive account on how to interpret an electrocardiogram.

Good Luck!

RECOMMENDED READING LIST

1. Shorter Books which may be useful for Revision

Use **one** of these three:
Lecture Notes on Clinical Medicine
D Rubenstein and D Wayne, Blackwell Scientific Publications, 1997

Oxford Handbook of Clinical Medicine
R A Hope and J M Longmore, Oxford University Press, 1998

Essential Medicine
A E Read and J V Jones, Churchill Livingstone, 1998

Both of these are also worth reading:
Oxford Handbook of Clinical Specialities
J A B Collier, J M Longmore and T J Hodgetts, Oxford University Press, 4th edition 1995

Essential Paediatrics
D Hull and D I Johnston, Churchill Livingstone (also available as an International Student Edition)

2. Books which are too long or detailed for revision but should be useful for reference

Acute Medicine
D C Sprigings and J B Chambers, Blackwell Scientific Publications, 2nd edition 1995.

Medical Emergencies – Diagnosis and Management
R Robinson and R B Stott, Butterworth Heinemann, 6th edition 1993

Clinical Medicine
P J Kumar and M L Clark, Balliere Tindall, 1998

Textbook of Medicine
R Souhami and J Moxham, Churchill Livingstone, 1997

Lecture Notes on General Surgery
H Ellis and R Calne, Blackwell Scientific Publications, 1998

Recommended Reading List

Handbook of General Surgery
P G Bevan and I A Donovan, Blackwell Scientific Publications, 1992

Concise System of Orthopaedics and Fractures
A G Apley and L Solomon, Butterworth Heinemann, 2nd edition 1994

Lecture Notes on Orthopaedics and Fractures
T Duckworth, Blackwell Scientific Publications, 3rd edition 1995

Lecture Notes on Gynaecology
G Chamberlain and J Malvern, Blackwell Scientific Publications, 1996

Gynaecology Illustrated
A D T Govan, C Hodge and R Callander, Churchill Livingstone, 4th edition 1993 (also available as an International Student Edition)

Lecture Notes on Obstetrics
G Chamberlain, M Pearce and P Hamilton, Blackwell Scientific Publications, 1996

Obstetrics Illustrated
A W F Miller and R Callander, Churchill Livingstone, 1997 (also available as an International Student Edition)

CONTRIBUTORS

Mr F Bindi   **MBBS (Lond), FRCS (Orth)**
Clinical Fellow, The Nuffield Orthopaedic Centre, Oxford

Ms D Eastwood   **FRCS**
Consultant Orthopaedic Surgeon, Honory Senior Lecturer, Royal Free Hospital/Royal National Orthopaedic Hospital

Dr B Gaspar   **BSc (Hons) MBBS MRCP (UK) MRCPCH PhD**
Clinical Lecturer in Immunology/Infectious Diseases, Institute of Child Health, University College, London

Dr N Maftei   **MD**
Senior House Officer, Aberdeen Royal Infirmary, Abderdeen

Dr S Mijatovic   **MD**
Senior House Officer, Frenchay Hospital, Bristol

Mr M K Oak   **MBBS ChM MPH FRCOG**
Consultant Obstetrician and Gynaecologist, Whipps Cross Hospital, London

Dr G Rees   **BM BCh MD MRCP PhD**
Wellcome Advanced Fellow, Institute of Neurology, University College London

Dr R Wasan   **BA MBBS MA MRCP FRCR**
Specialist Registrar in Radiology, St. George's Hospital, London

EMQ PRACTICE EXAMINATION

200 questions: time allowed 3 hours ✓

Theme: Abnormalities of water and electrolyte balance

Options

A   Addison's disease
B   Conn's syndrome
C   Diabetes insipidus
D   Renal tubular acidosis
E   Salmonella enteritis

For each presentation below, choose the SINGLE most likely diagnosis from the above list of options. Each option may be used once, more than once, or not at all.

	Na	K⁺	HCO₃⁻
1.	136	2.8	18
2.	149	2.6	30
3.	128	5.6	22
4.	130	2.5	8
5.	160	5.6	18

1

Theme: Abnormalities of acid-base balance

Options

A	Acute metabolic acidosis
B	Acute metabolic alkalosis
C	Acute respiratory acidosis
D	Acute respiratory alkalosis
E	Chronic respiratory acidosis

For each presentation below, choose the SINGLE most likely diagnosis from the above list of options. Each option may be used once, more than once, or not at all.

	pH	pCO_2	pO_2	HCO_3^-
6. A	7.20	2.2	11.8	12
7. B	7.64	5.4	12	38
8. C	7.20	8	5.8	24
9. D	7.62	1.8	13	19
10. E	7.28	7.8	6.2	33

Theme: Shortness of breath

Options

A	Anticoagulation	G	Rapid dehydration with
B	Chest drainage		normal saline
C	Correction of acidosis with intravenous bicarbonate	H	Re-breathing or sedation with benzodiazepine
D	Intravenous antibiotics (in combination with corticosteroids)	I	Thrombolysis with e.g. streptokinase
		J	Treatment with anti-malarial drugs (e.g. quinine)
E	Intravenous insulin		
F	Pain relief e.g. with non-steroidal anti-inflammatory drugs (NSAIDs)		

For each presentation below, choose the SINGLE most appropriate treatment from the above list of options. Each option may be used once, more than once, or not at all.

11. A 34-year-old man has suddenly developed dyspnoea (respiratory rate 42 breaths per minute) after return from a prolonged holiday in Thailand. His pulse oximetry reading is 80%, but you are not able to detect any abnormalities over the lungs.

12. A 50-year-old man has developed mild dyspnoea and positional chest pain, mainly lying flat. His electrocardiogram shows ST segment elevations in most leads. *pericarditis*

13. A 23-year-old woman is admitted with severe shortness of breath. Her respiratory rate is 48 breaths per minute. (Blood gas results: pH 7.52, pO_2 14 kPa, pCO_2 2.0 kPa)

14. A 20-year-old patient with non-insulin dependent diabetes has become progressively breathless over the last 24 hours. His pH is 7.2 and his pCO_2 2.2 kPa. The blood glucose concentration is 34 mmol/l.

15. A 26-year-old drug addict complains about severe shortness of breath for three days. The symptoms have developed gradually. Physical examination of his chest is normal, but his pulse oximetry readings are low (65–70% on air).

Theme: Findings on physical examination

Options

A	Cardiomyopathy	E	Multiple sclerosis
B	Holmes-Adie syndrome	F	Myasthenia gravis
C	Infectious polyneuritis	G	Pericardial disease
D	Intra-thoracic malignancy	H	Pulmonary valve stenosis

For each presentation below, choose the SINGLE most likely diagnosis from the above list of options. Each option may be used once, more than once, or not at all.

16. Increasing swelling of the face and neck.

17. The jugular venous pressure increases with inspiration.

18. Weakness in both legs with absent reflexes.

19. Pulsating liver

20. Dilated right pupil with poor light reaction and missing ankle jerks.

Theme: Basic differential diagnosis and treatment of emergencies

Options

A	Acute myocardial infarction	F	Pneumonia
B	Acute pulmonary oedema	G	Pneumothorax
C	Cardiogenic shock	H	Pulmonary embolism
D	Epileptic fit	I	Septic shock
E	Occult internal haemorrhage		

For each presentation below, choose the SINGLE most likely diagnosis from the above list of options. Each option may be used once, more than once, or not at all.

21. A 30-year-old woman has been unwell for six hours. Her vital signs are: pulse 130/min, BP 100/60 mmHg, temperature 40 °C, respiratory rate 44 breaths/min.

22. A 76-year-old man has collapsed in the street. His vital signs are: pulse 180/min, BP 60/? mmHg, temperature 36 °C, respiratory rate 29 breaths/min.

23. A 50-year-old builder develops severe dyspnoea and chest pain. His vital signs are: pulse 100/min, BP 240/160 mmHg, temperature 36 °C, respiratory rate 32 breaths/min.

24. An 18-year-old nanny has become increasingly drowsy and deliriant. She was well the day before admission. Her vital signs are: pulse 100/min, BP 50/? mmHg, temperature 39.5 °C, respiratory rate 26 breaths/min. There is a rash over her lower legs.

25. A 63-year-old heavy smoker has suddenly collapsed at home. His vital signs are: pulse 130 /min, BP 40/? mmHg, temperature 36 °C, respiratory rate 30 breaths/min. There are no neurological deficits; electrocardiogram and chest X-ray are normal.

Theme: Causes of headache

Options

A	Cluster headache	G	Metastatic disease
B	Extradural haemorrhage	H	Migraine
C	Giant cell arteritis	I	Subarachnoid haemorrhage
D	Glioblastoma multiforme	J	Subdural haematoma
E	Meningeoma	K	Tension headache
F	Meningitis	L	Trigeminal neuralgia

For each presentation below, choose the SINGLE most likely diagnosis from the above list of options. Each option may be used once, more than once, or not at all.

26. An elderly man complains of headache and progressive confusion over the past four months. CT scan of the brain reveals an irregularly enhancing mass in the left parietal lobe.

27. A previously fit and healthy 29-year-old man complains of sudden onset of severe headache, associated with nausea and vomiting. On examination he is drowsy (Glasgow Coma Scale (GCS) 9/15) and he has neck stiffness.

28. A 78-year-old man complains of headache and pain on chewing for three weeks. He has lost 10 kg in weight. His investigation results show a mild anaemia (Hb 11g/dl) and an ESR of 100 mm after one hour.

29. An 11-year-old girl is complaining of sudden-onset headache, nausea and vomiting. Her temperature is 40 °C.

30. A 36-year-old businessman has suffered from recurrent headaches for the last 4 months. He describes the headache 'to be like a very tight band around the head'.

Theme: Haematuria in children

Options

A	Acute glomerulonephritis
B	Benign recurrent haematuria
C	Haemolytic uraemic syndrome
D	Nephroblastoma
E	Renal venous thrombosis
F	Urinary tract infection

For each clinical scenario below, select the MOST likely cause of haematuria from the above list of options. Each option may be used once, more than once, or not at all.

31. A four-year-old child has an upper respiratory tract infection followed two weeks later by haematuria associated with oliguria and periorbital oedema.

32. A three-year-old girl has itching, frequency and pain on urination.

33. A child of four months presents with an abdominal mass and investigation shows displacement of the right kidney and there is microscopic haematuria.

34. A six-year-old has a number of episodes of painless macroscopic haematuria, with no evidence of a UTI and a normal IVU.

Theme: Electrocardiography

Options

A	Dominant QRS deflection negative in lead I
B	Dominant QRS deflection positive in lead I and negative in leads II and III
C	Dominant QRS deflection positive in leads I and II
D	High T waves (more than 2/3 of corresponding R waves)
E	Loss of R waves in lead V1
F	QT time prolonged
G	QT time shortened

For each presentation below, choose the SINGLE most likely diagnosis from the above list of options. Each option may be used once, more than once, or not at all.

35. Left axis deviation

36. Right axis deviation

37. Normal electrocardiographic axis

38. Hypokalaemia

39. Hypocalcaemia

40. Hyperkalaemia

Theme: Utero-vaginal prolapse

Options

A	Complete/III degree utero-vaginal prolapse
B	Manchester repair
C	No option applies
D	Ring or Smith's shelf and shaft pessary
E	This is a common complication after hysterectomy

For each presentation below, choose the SINGLE most likely diagnosis from the above list of options. Each option may be used once, more than once, or not at all.

41. Associated with urinary incontinence.

42. Method of choice in women who have not completed their family.

43. Procidentia

44. Ideal for elderly women with high anaesthetic risk.

45. Vault prolapse

Theme: Investigation of trauma

Options

A	Chest X-ray	E	MRI thoraco-lumbar spine
B	CT head scan	F	Shoulder X-ray
C	Lateral cervical spine X-ray	G	Skull X-ray
D	Lumbar spine X-ray	H	Ultrasound scan abdomen

Match the following symptoms and signs below to the SINGLE most helpful investigation from the above list. Each option may be used once, more than once, or not at all.

46. A 32-year-old boxer who complains of left-sided weakness 24 hours after a boxing match.

47. A 19-year-old man who has sustained stab wounds to his abdomen and trunk. His respiratory rate is 23 breaths/min, his breath sounds appear normal but his pulse is 142/min and his BP is only 80/40 mmHg.

48. A 47-year-old woman complains of left shoulder and neck pain after having fallen off her bicycle. She has a graze on her forehead and also complains of tingling in her left ring and little fingers (digits IV and V).

49. A 27-year-old motorcyclist has been involved in an accident and complains of loss of sensation below the umbilicus and paralysis of both legs. His BP is 80/50 mmHg with a pulse rate of 72/min.

50. A 54-year-old roofer complains of lower back pain radiating into the right leg having fallen from a scaffold. He has no loss of power or sensation when examined.

Theme: The painful red eye

Options

A	Acute cellulitis	G	Ulcerative keratitis
B	Chronic open angle glaucoma	H	Urgent referral to eye surgeon
C	Closed angle glaucoma	I	Uveitis
D	Foreign body	J	Viral conjunctivitis
E	Intra-ocular tumour	K	Vitreous haemorrhage
F	Subconjunctival haemorrhage		

For each case below, choose the SINGLE most appropriate diagnosis from the above list of options. Each option may be used once, more than once, or not at all.

51. A 36-year-old man complains about sudden-onset pain in the right eye, blurred vision and profuse lacrimation. On examination the eye is red and his visual acuity is not significantly reduced. Additionally, he complains about back pain and stiffness in his lower spine.

52. After a prolonged and difficult labour a 26-year-old woman has successfully delivered a large baby (4330 grams) per vaginam. The midwife is concerned that the mother has developed red eyes.

53. A 24-year-old man presents to his GP complaining of burning, itching eyes and lacrimation. On examination you find mild erythema in both eyes, but visual acuity is normal. He is also complaining about painful eye movements.

54. A 65-year-old man complains about sudden-onset left eye pain, which started while driving his car. On examination the eye is red and his visual acuity is reduced. He claims to see a 'halo' around lights and describes his visual loss as 'looking through frosted glass'.

55. A newborn baby (12 days old) has developed a red left eye with purulent discharge.

56. A 48-year-old man with a recent injury of his left cheek was admitted with marked left-sided periorbital swelling, red eye and blurred vision. He has high fever and is drowsy.

Theme: Childhood investigations

Options

A	Bone marrow aspirate	F	Lung biopsy
B	Brain biopsy	G	Muscle biopsy
C	Cardiac biopsy	H	Rectal biopsy
D	Jejunal biopsy	I	Splenic aspirate
E	Liver biopsy		

Which biopsy/investigation from the options listed above would you use to diagnose the following conditions? Each option may be used once, more than once, or not at all.

57. Duchenne's muscular dystrophy

58. Leishmaniasis

59. Subacute Sclerosing Panencephalitis (SSPE)

60. Hirschsprung's disease

Theme: Multiple trauma

Options

A   Fractured os calcis and thoraco-lumbar vertebrae
B   Fractured pelvis, femur and cervical spine
C   Fractured right humerus, right femur and pelvis
D   Head/facial injury, fractured sternum, tibial fractures
E   Respiratory distress and facial burns

Match the following patients to the SINGLE most likely pattern of injury from the options listed above. Each option may be used once, more than once, or not at all.

61.   A 37-year-old driver of a car struck by a van on the driver's side.

62.   A 25-year-old roofer falling 7 metres to the ground, landing feet first.

63.   A 43-year-old man involved in an explosion at a petro-chemical plant.

64.   The driver of a car involved in a head-on collision whilst not wearing a seat belt.

65.   A 19-year-old motorcyclist thrown 19 metres from his motorbike.

Theme: The painful hip in children

Options

A   Developmental dysplasia of the hip (CDH)
B   Irritable hip syndrome
C   Osteomyelitis
D   Perthes' disease
E   Septic arthritis
F   Slipped upper femoral epiphysis (SUFE)

Match the following symptoms and signs listed below with the SINGLE most likely condition from the options above. Each option may be used once, more than once, or not at all.

66.   A six-year-old boy complains of intermittent hip pain for several months. Haematological investigations are normal. X-rays show flattening of the femoral head.

67.   A two-year-old girl with a one-day history of increasing hip pain has become unable to weight bear. Her WCC is 22/fl, with an ESR of 88 mm/hour and a CRP of 300 mg/l. A radiograph of the hip shows a widened joint space.

68.   A 12-year-old boy with left groin pain for 6 weeks is noticed to stand with the left leg externally rotated. Examination reveals negligible internal rotation of the hip.

69.   A four-year-old boy complains of right hip pain a few days following an upper respiratory tract infection. Blood tests are as follows: WCC=12/fl, ESR=10 mm/hour and CRP=2 mg/l.

70.   A five-year-old girl complains of progressively increasing severe pain in her left hip and upper leg for 6 days. She is able to walk but limps visibly. Blood tests are as follows: WCC=19/fl, ESR 72 mm/hour and CRP 94 mg/l. X-rays and ultrasound scans of the hip are normal.

Theme: *Cervical disc prolapse*

Options

A	C5 nerve root
B	C6 nerve root
C	C7 nerve root
D	C8 nerve root
E	T1 nerve root

Altered sensation or paraesthesia over the following areas listed below suggests involvement of which of the nerve roots from the above list of options? Each option may be used once, more than once, or not at all.

71. Thumb

72. Outer forearm

73. Upper outer arm

74. Middle finger

75. Little finger

Theme: Jaundice in childhood

Options

A	ABO incompatibility	F	Galactosaemia
B	Biliary atresia	G	Gilbert's syndrome
C	Breast milk jaundice	H	Glucose-6-phospho-
D	Congenital toxoplasma		diesterase deficiency
	infection	I	Hereditary spherocytosis
E	Crigler-Najjar syndrome		

For the list of scenarios below select the correct cause from the options above. Each option may be used once, more than once, or not at all.

76. A newborn develops an unconjugated hyperbilirubinaemia 12 hours after birth associated with a severe metabolic acidosis.

77. An infant is jaundiced at birth and is found on examination to have a distended abdomen with organomegaly. The infant also has convulsions.

78. A newborn develops a progressive conjugated hyperbilirubinaemia with pale stools and dark urine.

79. A full-term infant develops jaundice on day three, which continues for two weeks. The hyperbilirubinaemia is unconjugated, there is no derangement of other liver function tests and the child remains clinically well.

Theme: Treatment of femoral fractures

Options

A	Dynamic hip screw (DHS)	F	Open reduction and internal fixation (ORIF)
B	Gallows traction		
C	Hemiarthroplasty	G	Skeletal traction
D	Intramedullary nailing	H	Total hip replacement (THR)
E	Multiple cannulated hip screws		

Choose the MOST appropriate form of treatment from the above list of options for each of the following fractures. Each option may be used once, more than once, or not at all.

80. A 78-year-old lady with a displaced subcapital (Garden IV) fracture of the left femoral neck.

81. A 24-year-old motorcyclist with a closed fracture of the right femoral shaft.

82. A nine-month-old child with a spiral fracture of the femoral shaft.

83. A 57-year-old lady with an undisplaced fracture of the right femoral neck.

84. An 83-year-old lady with a displaced intertrochanteric fracture.

Theme: Management of infertility

Options

A	Bacteriological examination of urine
B	Day 21 progesterone
C	Semen analysis
D	Tubal patency test
E	Wait and see

For each presentation below, choose the SINGLE most likely diagnosis from the above list of options. Each option may be used once, more than once, or not at all.

85. A couple aged 25 years have been trying for a baby for six months.

86. Useful in determining ovulation.

87. An essential investigation for all heterosexual infertile couples.

88. This investigation is of little value.

89. Is an essential investigation of the female partner.

Theme: Back pain

Options

A	Bony metastasis	F	Mechanical back pain
B	Central disc prolapse	G	Osteoporotic vertebral
C	Dissecting abdominal aortic		body crush fracture
	aneurysm	H	Spinal stenosis
D	L1–L2 disc prolapse	I	Spinal tuberculosis
E	L4–L5 disc prolapse		

For each of the following clinical pictures choose the MOST likely diagnosis from the above list of options. Each option may be used once, more than once, or not all.

90. A 33-year-old male company director complains of intermittent lower back pain in the absence of any neurological symptoms or signs. Radiographs are normal.

91. A 43-year-old woman complains of sudden onset lower back pain radiating down the left leg as far as the heel. She has paraesthesiae over the lateral aspect of the left lower leg and foot. Examination reveals straight leg raising (SLR) limited to 20 degrees with altered sensation in the above distribution.

92. A 68-year-old woman complains of bilateral buttock and thigh pain associated with back pain after walking 200 metres; sitting down relieves the pain. She does not experience any symptoms at rest. Examination of the back is unremarkable.

93. A 28-year-old woman has severe lower back pain; she is incontinent of urine. Examination reveals loss of sensation over the perineum and straight leg raise is limited bilaterally.

94. A 72-year-old man complains of severe back pain not responding to rest. He is unable to sleep and has lost 6 Kg in weight over the last two months. Examination reveals some tenderness in the lumbar region but no neurological abnormalities.

Theme: Short stature in children

Options

A	Achondroplasia	F	Klinefelter's syndrome
B	Congenital hypothyroidism	G	Noonan's syndrome
C	Down's syndrome	H	Russell-Silver syndrome
D	Growth hormone deficiency	I	Turner's syndrome
E	Hypopituitarism		

For each child listed below choose the MOST likely cause of short stature from the options listed above. Each option may be used once, more than once, or not at all.

95. A child with an abnormally sized head and predominant shortening of the proximal upper and lower limbs.

96. A six-year-old boy with webbing of the neck, cubitus valgus and congenital heart disease.

97. A seven-year-old boy previously treated with cranial irradiation for a brain tumour has recurrent episodes of hypoglycaemia.

98. A two year-old with poor motor and speech development, large tongue and umbilical hernia.

Theme: Urinary incontinence

Options

A   Detrusor instability
B   Genuine stress incontinence
C   None of the above
D   Retention with overflow
E   Urinary fistula

For each presentation below, choose the SINGLE most likely diagnosis from the above list of options. Each option may be used once, more than once, or not at all.

99. History of dysuria, frequency and foul smelling urine.

100. History of urgency and frequency of micturition and inability to hold urine as soon as the urge to pass urine is felt.

101. History of leakage of small amounts of urine following an operation for stress incontinence.

102. Urinary incontinence when intra-abdominal pressure is raised, e.g. on coughing and sneezing.

103. Continuous leak of small quantity of urine following Wertheim's hysterectomy for stage Ib carcinoma of the cervix.

Theme: Chest trauma

Options

A	Abdominal ultrasound	E	MRI scan chest
B	Chest drain	F	MRI scanning
C	Chest radiograph	G	Needle thoracocentesis
D	Computed tomography	H	Pericardiocentesis

For each of the following scenarios, choose the MOST appropriate investigation from the above list of options. Each option may be used once, more than once, or not at all.

104. A 35-year-old man has been stabbed in the left lower chest from behind with a 5 centimetre long blade. His BP is 80/60 mmHg with a pulse of 110/min. He has normal breath sounds and no evidence of pneumothorax on X-ray.

C

105. A 20-year-old horse rider has sustained a crush injury to the chest when her horse landed on her during a fall. On examination you find tenderness on the right side of her chest with decreased breath sounds and dullness to percussion. Her vital signs are a pulse of 110/min and BP is 100/80 mmHg.

G

106. A 32-year-old driver of a car involved in a head on collision has evidence of blunt chest trauma to the sternum area. His BP is 90/60 mmHg with a pulse of 120/min. He has prominent neck veins and muffled heart sounds. Chest X-ray is normal.

107. A 27-year-old motorcyclist involved in a road traffic accident (RTA) complains of difficulty in breathing. He has a respiratory rate of 40 breaths/min, decreased chest movements and air entry on the right along with hyper-resonance on percussion. His pulse oximeter readings are around 80% on oxygen.

B

108. A 37-year-old man was involved in a high speed RTA. He is unconscious with evidence of bruising across his chest. Despite intravenous fluid replacement with 4 litres of Hartmann's solution, he remains hypotensive. His X-ray shows a widened mediastinum.

H

Theme: Developmental milestones of children

Options

A	6 weeks
B	6 months
C	1 year
D	2 years
E	3 years
F	5 years

From the above options select the age at which you would expect a normal child to achieve the following developmental stages listed below? Each option may be used once, more than once, or not at all.

C **109.** Sitting unaided *B*

A **110.** Smiling

D **111.** Walks up stairs

112. Dry by day *E*

C **113.** Cruising around furniture

Theme: Vaccines

Options

A	Hib
B	Mantoux
C	Pneumovax
D	Rubella
E	Salk polio
F	Tetanus

For each description of vaccine type given below, choose the MOST likely vaccine from the above list. Each option may be used once, more than once, or not at all.

114. Killed

115. Conjugate

116. Live

117. Polysaccharide

Theme: Congenital infections in childhood

Options

A   Congenital CMV infection
B   Congenital Herpes simplex infection
C   Congenital parvovirus
D   Congenital rubella
E   Congenital syphilis
F   Congenital toxoplasmosis

Which congenital infection listed in the options above is MOST likely in the following clinical cases? Each option may be used once, more than once, or not at all.

118. A newborn child with thrombocytopenia, hepatosplenomegaly, retinitis and periventricular calcification on CT scan of the head.

119. A newborn girl with hepatosplenomegaly, chorioretinitis, and tram-like calcifications on CT scan of the head.

120. A newborn boy with skeletal changes suggestive of recurrent periostitis, a bony prominence of the head and a saddle nose.

121. A stillborn child with non-immune (i.e. compatible rhesus constellation) hydrops fetalis.

Theme: Abnormal smear

Options

A	Colposcopy is indicated
B	Cytobrush technique is indicated
C	Dyskaryosis
D	Dysplasia
E	May be a false positive result

For each presentation below, choose the SINGLE most likely diagnosis from the above list of options. Each option may be used once, more than once, or not at all.

122. Must be used in a woman in whom previous colposcopy was incomplete.

123. Repeat smear test necessary in the first instance.

124. Within three months from the end of pregnancy.

125. This is a histological diagnosis.

126. With two or more inadequate smears.

Theme: Increased susceptibility to infection

Options

A	Bruton's agamma-globulinaemia
B	Chédiak-Higashi syndrome
C	Chronic granulomatous disease
D	Complement deficiency
E	Hyper IgE syndrome
F	IgA deficiency
G	Severe combined immunodeficiency

Susceptibility to which infections listed below is MOST characteristic of the above immunodeficiency syndromes. Each option may be used once, more than once or not all.

127. Recurrent *Neisseria meningitidis* infection

128. *Pneumocystis carinii* pneumonitis

129. Aspergillus infection

130. Staphylococcal skin abscesses

Theme: Complications of total hip replacement (THR)

Options

A	Anterior dislocation	E	Deep vein thrombosis (DVT)
B	Cellulitis	F	Haematoma
C	Chest infection	G	Posterior dislocation
D	Deep infection	H	Pulmonary embolism (PE)

Choose the MOST likely diagnosis from the above list of options for each of the following clinical presentations. Each option may be used once, more than once, or not at all.

131. A 73-year-old man complains of swelling and discoloration of the right leg seven days after a right THR. He has tenderness behind the right knee on palpation.

132. An 81-year-old lady develops a pyrexia of 38 °C three weeks after her left THR. Her wound is oozing and her blood tests reveal a CRP of 150 mg/l and an ESR of 96 mm/hour.

133. A 67-year-old lady develops swelling and bruising of the left thigh four days after her left THR. Blood tests are normal.

134. A 77-year-old man develops sudden chest pain and breathlessness five days after his left THR. His pulse oximetry readings are 82% on air.

135. A 75-year-old lady develops sudden severe pain in her right hip whilst sitting down three weeks after her right THR. She is unable to stand and her right leg is internally rotated, flexed and adducted at the hip.

Theme: Skin disease in children

Options

A	Erythema chronicum migrans	E	Exanthema subitum
B	Erythema infectiosum	F	Purpura fulminans
C	Erythema multiforme	G	Tinea corporis
D	Erythema nodosum		

For the clinical scenarios listed below choose the condition MOST associated from the above list of options. Each option may be used once, more than once or not at all.

136. A nine-month-old child is non-specifically unwell for three days with a fever. The rash subsides and the child breaks out in a maculo-papular rash over its body.

137. Following a course of Septrin for a bacterial infection, a five-year-old child breaks out in a widespread macular rash with target lesions.

138. A four-year-old boy has a runny nose and mild fever and develops bright red cheeks and reticular rash on the forearms.

139. Following a tick bite on holiday in a forested area, a seven-year-old boy develops an erythematous macule at the site of the bite which then spreads into an annular lesion with a clear central area.

Theme: Drugs in childhood

Options

A	Aminophylline	F	Cefotaxime
B	Aspirin	G	Cisapride
C	Azithromycin	H	Isoniazid
D	Benzylpenicillin	I	Tetracyclines
E	Brufen		

For the list of scenarios below select the correct drug from the options above. Each option may be used once, more than once, or not at all.

140. Is recommended as first line empirical therapy in bacterial meningitis where the cause of infection is not known.

141. Is not recommended for analgesic or antipyretic use in children under 12 years of age due to the risk of Reye's syndrome.

142. Causes arrhythmias in association with antifungal agents.

143. Should not be given to children under 12 years of age as it can cause staining and malformation of teeth.

Theme: Genetic defects

Options

A	Angelman's syndrome	E	Klinefelter's syndrome
B	Beckwith-Wiedemann syndrome	F	Noonan's syndrome
		G	Russell-Silver syndrome
C	Down's syndrome	H	Turner's syndrome
D	Edward's syndrome		

Choose the MOST likely genetic defect from the list of options above for each clinical scenario listed below. Each option may be used once, more than once, or not at all?

144. A newborn male who is hypotonic and noted to have brachycephaly and recurrent vomiting due to duodenal atresia.

145. A 14-year-old girl of normal intelligence who is short for her age and has not yet started to menstruate.

146. A small for dates newborn with small chin, severe mental retardation and abnormally shaped soles of the feet.

147. A five-year-old girl with short stature and hypertrophy of her left-sided limbs and mild mental retardation.

Theme: Intra-uterine contraceptive device (IUCD)

Options

A	Antibiotic therapy and remove IUCD
B	Contraindicated
C	IUCD should be inserted after the next period
D	Remove IUCD and offer alternative contraception
E	Suspect ectopic pregnancy – refer to early pregnancy assessment unit

For each patient below choose the MOST appropriate option from the list above. Each option may be used once, more than once, or not at all.

148. A 25-year-old woman is complaining of persistent lower abdominal pain and irregular vaginal bleeding since the insertion of an IUCD six months ago.

149. A 32-year-old woman who had an IUCD inserted three weeks ago is complaining of severe abdominal pain. On examination: pulse 92/min, temp 37.7 °C; the abdomen is tender but there is no rigidity or guarding.

150. A 27-year-old woman has come to your family planning clinic requesting insertion of an IUCD. Her last menstrual period was three weeks ago.

151. A woman in her early twenties presents with left iliac fossa pain and vaginal bleeding for three days. An IUCD was inserted three months ago and her last normal period was five weeks ago.

152. A woman in her late twenties with a history of pelvic inflammatory disease was reported to have pelvic adhesions at laparoscopy six months ago and is requesting an IUCD for contraception.

Theme: Ankle injuries

Options

A	Elastic bandage and physiotherapy
B	External fixation
C	External fixation and wound débridement
D	Manipulation under anaesthesia (MUA) and POP application
E	Open reduction and internal fixation (ORIF)
F	Plaster of Paris (POP) immobilisation
G	Suture repair

Choose the MOST appropriate form of treatment from the list of options above for each of the following clinical conditions. Each option may be used once, more than once or not at all.

153. A 26-year-old man complains of sudden onset pain at the back of his heel and calf whilst playing squash. He has calf tenderness and is unable to stand on his toes; X-rays are normal.

154. A 54-year-old woman sustains a twisting injury to the left ankle whilst stepping off a kitchen ladder. She has swelling and tenderness over the lateral aspect of the ankle. X-rays show an undisplaced fracture of the distal fibula.

155. A 23-year-old motorcyclist involved in a RTA has a compound (open) fracture of the left tibia with extension into the ankle joint.

156. A 31-year-old footballer sustains an injury to the right ankle in a tackle. There is swelling and tenderness over both medial and lateral aspects of the ankle. X-rays show a displaced fracture of the distal fibula (Weber type C) with evidence of talar shift.

157. A 43-year-old window cleaner falls off a ladder injuring his left heel. X-rays confirm an extra-articular fracture of the calcaneum.

Theme: Investigations of postmenopausal bleeding

Options

A   Full blood count
B   None of the above
C   Pipelle biopsy
D   Referral to gynaecology clinic
E   Transvaginal ultrasound scan
F   Vulval biopsy

For each presentation below, choose the SINGLE most likely diagnosis from the above list of options. Each option may be used once, more than once, or not at all.

158. Postmenopausal woman complaining of pruritus vulvae.

159. A 50-year-old woman on cyclical hormone replacement therapy complains of irregular vaginal bleeding.

160. An episode of vaginal bleeding ten years after the menopause.

161. A 60-year-old woman complaining of labial ulceration and bleeding.

162. Is of little value in the management of postmenopausal bleeding.

Theme: Contraception

Options

A   Associated with pelvic pain
B   Break through bleeding is a common side-effect
C   Consider ectopic pregnancy
D   Is associated with irregular bleeding
E   Suitable in a stable relationship

For each presentation below, choose the SINGLE most likely diagnosis from the above list of options. Each option may be used once, more than once, or not at all.

163. Progesterone contraceptives

164. Intrauterine contraceptive devices

165. Biphasic pill

166. History of irregular period and pelvic pain

167. Rhythm method

Theme: Investigations of pruritus vulvae

Options

A	Creatinine clearance
B	Glucose tolerance test
C	High vaginal swab
D	None of the listed options
E	Vulval biopsy

For each presentation below, choose the SINGLE most likely diagnosis from the above list of options. Each option may be used once, more than once, or not at all.

168. Must be done in a woman with associated history of vaginal discharge.

169. A woman with a history of postmenopausal bleeding.

170. This investigation is unnecessary.

171. A 45-year-old woman with associated vulval ulceration.

172. In a 38-year-old woman with gestational diabetes mellitus in her three pregnancies.

Theme Causes of amenorrhoea

Options

A   Drug side-effect
B   Imperforate hymen
C   Likely to be premature menopause
D   Post pill amenorrhoea
E   Primary amenorrhoea

For each presentation below, choose the SINGLE most likely diagnosis from the above list of options. Each option may be used once, more than once, or not at all.

173. A 34-year-old woman being treated for endometriosis.

174. A 32-year-old woman with a history of hot flushes.

175. A 14-year-old girl who is experiencing cyclical pelvic and vaginal pain but no period.

176. A 17-year-old girl who has had only withdrawal bleeds.

177. A 24-year-old woman has recently discontinued contraceptive precaution.

Theme: Vaginal discharge

Options

A   A common cause in pre-pubertal girls
B   Can be diagnosed clinically
C   Is more common with systemic antibiotic treatment, diabetes and in pregnancy
D   This has no diagnostic value
E   Treat with diathermy

For each presentation below, choose the SINGLE most likely diagnosis or treatment from the above list of options. Each option may be used once, more than once, or not at all.

178. Persistent vaginal discharge with cervical erosion

179. Candidiasis

180. Trichomonas

181. Foreign body in the vagina

182. Liver function test

Theme: The painful knee

Options

A	Anterior knee pain in a 15-year-old gymnast with no history of trauma
B	Giving way and intermittent swelling
C	Intermittent locking and swelling in a patient with osteochondritis dissecans
D	Pain along the medial joint line, swelling and inability to extend the joint fully
E	Pain over the proximal tibia associated with a tender swelling

Match the conditions listed below to the SINGLE most likely clinical picture from the options above. Each option may be used once, more than once, or not at all.

183. Anterior cruciate ligament rupture

184. Loose body

185. Chondromalacia patellae

186. Medial meniscus tear

187. Osgood Schlatter's disease

Theme: Viral infections in childhood

Options

A	Adenovirus	F	Molluscum contagiosum
B	Cytomegalovirus	G	Mumps
C	ECHO virus	H	Rotavirus
D	Enterovirus		
E	Epstein-Barr virus		

For each group of symptoms listed below, select the MOST likely causative agent from the list of options above. Each option may be used once, more than once, or not at all.

188. A four-month-old child of an HIV positive mother is perfectly well until he develops a cough and tachypnoea. He soon requires ventilation and the chest X-ray shows bilateral pneumonitis.

189. A ten-year-old boy develops high fever with generalised lymphadenopathy and hepatosplenomegaly four weeks after he has a liver transplant.

190. An 18-month-old boy from a travelling family is admitted with unilateral parotid swelling and has signs of meningism.

191. A three-year-old has a crop of raised discrete lesions with umbilicated centres on his abdomen. They persist for several months but the child remains well.

Theme: *Causes of dementia*

Options

A	Alzheimer's disease	E	Hypothyroidism
B	Creutzfeldt-Jacob disease	F	Post-ictal confusion
C	Depression	G	Wernicke's encephalopathy
D	Huntington's disease		

For each patient with memory loss below, select the MOST likely diagnosis from the above list of options. Each option may be used once, more than once or not at all.

192. A 43-year-old unmarried woman has had poor memory and sleep disturbance for the last three weeks. She has been living alone after recently moving to the United Kingdom. Neurologic examination is normal.

193. A 65-year-old man gives a six-month history of forgetfulness and progressively mislaying items around the home. His wife reports he occasionally gets lost when out walking around their neighbourhood. Neurological examination is unremarkable.

194. A 36-year-old woman is brought to hospital having being found unconscious at home after falling down the stairs. She cannot remember anything about the episode, is mildly disoriented and has broken her wrist. Neurologic examination is otherwise unremarkable.

195. A 32-year-old homeless woman is brought to hospital complaining of memory loss. She is disoriented in space and time, has gait ataxia and a right sixth nerve palsy. A CT (head) is normal.

196. A 24-year-old man complains of low mood and sleep disturbance for the last two months. In the last two weeks he reports difficulty remembering the names of familiar objects and difficulty writing. Myoclonus in the upper limbs is noted on examination.

Theme: Drug management of psychiatric disease

Options

A	Amitriptyline	E	Chlorpromazine
B	Atropine	F	Lithium carbonate
C	Carbamazepine	G	Lorazepam
D	Chlordiazepoxide		

For each patient below, select the MOST appropriate drug that should be administered from the above list of options. Each option may be used once, more than once or not at all.

197. A 63-year-old man presents in an agitated state with confusion and visual hallucinations that terrify him. He has pyrexia, tremor and tachycardia and is sweating profusely. He has previously been admitted repeatedly with symptoms associated with chronic alcoholism.

198. A 30-year-old woman is brought to Casualty in an agitated and distractable state. She is in an expansive euphoric mood and will not stop talking. Her friends report that her agitated and excitable behavior has recently resulted in dismissal from her job.

199. An 83-year old man gives a three-month history of increasing insomnia, fatigue and difficulty concentrating. He has lost interest in daily activities and feels a burden on his family.

200. The police bring a 45-year-old man to Casualty after threatening staff at a nearby store. He has prominent third-person auditory hallucinations and states that the Queen of England, via a radio-transmitter implanted in his teeth, controls his actions.

EMQ PRACTICE EXAMINATION –
ANSWERS AND EXPLANATIONS

Theme: Abnormalities of water and electrolyte balance

1. **D**

   The hallmark of renal tubular acidosis is a mild metabolic acidosis with hypokalaemia. The normal range for serum bicarbonate concentration is 22 to 28 mmol/l. The low level suggests acidosis. The clinical picture is common after therapy with acetazolamide

2. **B**

   Conn's syndrome or primary hyperaldosteronism is a rare condition, but it is important as a cause of secondary arterial hypertension. The main clinical feature is hypertension without oedema and the combination of mild hypernatraemia with hypokalaemia.

3. **A**

   Addison's disease or adrenal failure is characterised by low blood pressure, skin and buccal pigmentation and the combination of hyponatraemia and mild hyperkalaemia.

4. **E**

   Severe diarrhoea results in metabolic acidosis due to bicarbonate loss and hypokalaemia (Remember: The bicarbonate content of bowel is approximately 80 mmol/l).

5. **C**

   Diabetes insipidus is due to ADH deficiency or lack/loss of renal ADH responsiveness. These patients lose predominately free water and present with polyuria and dehydration. Other causes of such electrolyte constellation are poor fluid intake or water loss due to fever/hyperventilation.

Theme: Abnormalities of acid-base balance

6. **A**

   Remember the normal values of blood gas analysis: pH 7.36–7.44; $pO_2 > 11$ kPa; pCO_2 4.6–5.5 kPa; Bicarbonate 22–28 mmol/l. The differential diagnosis follows a simple two step approach: if pH less than 7.36 ⇒ diagnose acidosis; if pCO_2 normal or low ⇒ diagnose metabolic acidosis.

7. **B**

   First step: pH > 7.44 ⇒ alkalosis
   Second step: pCO_2 normal or high ⇒ metabolic alkalosis.

8. **C**

   First step: pH < 7.36 ⇒ acidosis
   Second step: pCO_2 high ⇒ respiratory acidosis. The normal bicarbonate concentration makes an acute respiratory acidosis likely.

9. **D**

   First step: pH > 7.44 ⇒ alkalosis
   Second step: pCO_2 low ⇒ respiratory alkalosis.

10. **E**

    First step: pH < 7.36 ⇒ acidosis
    Second step: $pCO_2 > 5.5$ kPa ⇒ respiratory acidosis
    Third step: bicarbonate > 30 mmol/l ⇒ chronic respiratory alkalosis likely.

NB. In real life mixed acid-base disturbances are common which are best tackled with a nomogram (see Oxford Handbook of Clinical Medicine listed in the Recommended Reading List page xi).

Theme: Shortness of breath

11. **A**

The likely diagnosis is pulmonary embolism. Anticoagulation with a heparin is the accepted treatment.

12. **F**

The description is suggestive of pericarditis. Anticoagulation or thrombolysis is contraindicated, because it might cause haemopericardium and cardiac tamponade.

13. **H**

The diagnosis is hyperventilation syndrome. Re-breathing into a plastic bag is in most instances sufficient to relief the symptoms. The underlying problem is commonly an acute anxiety state and sedation with a benzodiazepine might be necessary.

14. **G**

Rehydration with normal saline has priority in diabetic ketoacidosis. The estimated fluid deficit in decompensated ketoacidosis is approximately 10% of body weight. Insulin treatment is the next step; correction with bicarbonate solution is not necessary and might be harmful.

15. **D**

Drug addicts are a high-risk group for contracting HIV. *Pneumocystis carinii* pneumonia is a common first manifestation of immunodeficiency. The treatment of this type of pneumonia consists of high dose co-trimoxazole and in severe cases corticosteroids are added.

Theme: Findings on physical examination

16. **D**

    The patient has superior vena cava syndrome. The most common cause is bronchial carcinoma. Metastatic spread into the mediastinal lymph glands causes mechanical flow obstruction of the superior vena cava. The clinical syndrome is characterised by swelling of the neck, head and arms.

17. **G**

    This clinical presentation is known as Kussmaul's sign. It is caused by pericardial tamponade or constriction.

18. **C**

    Infectious polyneuritis is the likely diagnosis from the option list.

19. **A**

    A pulsating liver is mostly due to tricuspid valve insufficiency. In dilated cardiomyopathy this is a common finding.

20. **B**

    Holmes-Adie syndrome is the correct answer. The exact pathology of the peripheral reflex loss is not known; the pupillary malfunction might be due to a defect in the ciliary ganglion.

Theme: Basic differential diagnosis and treatment of emergencies

21. F

The most likely diagnosis is pneumonia. The combination of fever and high respiratory rate is the typical clinical finding.

22. C

This gentleman has cardiogenic shock due to tachyarrhythmia, e.g. fast atrial fibrillation.

23. B

Acute pulmonary oedema due to hypertensive crisis is the correct diagnosis.

24. I

The young woman is in septic shock. The rash suggests meningo-coccal disease.

25. E

The normal electrocardiogram (see Appendix 3 page 89) and chest X-ray makes a cardiac cause of shock unlikely. Consider a sudden internal haemorrhage e.g. from leaking aortic aneurysm or perforated peptic ulcer.

Theme: Causes of headache

26. **D**
27. **I**
28. **C**
29. **F**
30. **K**

These are the classical description of the various headache types. The most common forms are tension and migranous headaches. Clinically a stepdown approach is necessary. First, exclude potentially serious diseases such as meningitis (fever and rash) and subarachnoid haemorrhages (sudden onset of severe headache in previously well person). The commonest type of intracranial malignancy is metastatic disease. However, single irregular lesions (such as in question 26) are mostly aggressive gliomas. Do not forget other causes of headaches such as sinusitis, osteoarthritis of the temporomandibular joint, tooth abcess and cluster headaches. The latter present mainly in middle-aged men with profuse lacrimation and pain around the eye.

Theme: Haematuria in children

31. A

In children acute glomerulonephritis often follows a sore throat or Upper Respiratory Tract Infection (URTI) and the causative organism is normally a Group A Streptococcus. The combination of haematuria, oliguria and periorbital oedema suggests nephritis. A raised ASOT would suggest that a streptococcal infection was the cause.

32. F

This describes the common features of a urinary tract infection (UTI). Diagnosis is made by examination and culture of the urine.

33. D

Nephroblastoma usually presents with abdominal distension and the finding of a mass in the abdomen. Haematuria is an uncommon but well recognised finding.

34. B

The lack of infection, a normal urinary tract and repeated episodes suggest a benign recurrent haematuria. The aetiology of this condition is unclear.

Theme: Electrocardiography

35. B

The electrocardiographic axis is easily determined from leads I and II. If the major QRS deflection is positive (upwards, R-wave) in lead I and II, the axis is normal. If it is only positive in lead I the diagnosis is left axis deviation and if it is negative in lead I the diagnosis is right axis deviation.

36. A

See answer above.

37. C

See answer 35.

38. F

Hypokalaemia and hypocalcaemia prolong the QT interval.

39. F

40. D

Hyperkalaemia can produce high T waves in electrocardiographic recordings. Other conditions are hyperacute myocardial infarction and it may also be found as a normal variant in young, fit adults.

NB. Refer to Appendix 3,
How to interpret the electrocardiogram pg 89

Theme: Utero-vaginal prolapse

41. **C**
42. **B**
43. **A**
44. **D**
45. **E**

The incidence of utero-vaginal prolapse is rising due to the ageing of our population. However, it is occasionally seen in young women and in these cases a Manchester repair is performed. Vault prolapse is common after a hysterectomy. The term procidentia means complete utero-vaginal prolapse. Ring or Smith shelf and shaft pessary is the preferred method of management in women who are a poor anaesthetic risk or who do not want an operation.

Theme: Investigation of trauma

46. B

This man probably has a subdural haemorrhage. A history of blows to the head and delayed onset of neurological symptoms should arouse suspicion. Considerable delay of clinical presentation in this condition is not unusual, as the bleeding is venous in origin.

47. H

This man is in circulatory shock. The likely cause is blood loss into the abdominal cavity. An ultrasound scan is a rapid and accurate way of identifying intra-peritoneal fluid. Peritoneal lavage as often quoted in older textbooks but is rarely indicated.

48. C

This lady's frontal graze is evidence of an axial compression injury to the neck. A cervical spine lateral X-ray will detect an abnormality with a sensitivity of 90%.

49. E

This man has spinal injuries with neurogenic shock i.e. hypotension in the presence of a normal pulse rate. The sensory deficit suggests a lower thoracic spine injury (umbilicus = T 10).

50. D

A fracture of a lumbar vertebra is the most likely diagnosis. In the absence of any neurological deficit a plain X-ray should be the first investigation. This will allow identification of the level of injury. Subsequently a CT scan or MRI may be required to assess the stability of the injured vertebra and integrity of the spinal canal.

Theme: The painful red eye

51. I

This is the classical description of a patient with ankylosing spondylitis. The X-ray of his lumbar spine is often unremarkable in the early stages of the disease. Bone scanning or special views of the ileosacral joints are methods to detect early disease.

52. F

Not an uncommon situation. Due to the high venous pressure when pushing down to expel the baby small vessels burst in the conjunctiva. No treatment is needed, but warn the mother that it might take a week or two before the redness in the eye clears up.

53. J

A viral conjunctivitis is the correct diagnosis. Viral infections often cause diffuse myalgia; pain with extreme eye movements is a common finding.

54. C

This is the classical description of acute closed angle glaucoma.

55. H

The diagnosis is ophthalmia neonatorum and an emergency. The child has to be admitted under the care of an eye surgeon and the disease has to be notified. A bacterial infection (especially sexually transmitted diseases such as gonorrhoea, chlamydia and staphylococcus) must be considered.

56. A

Periorbital cellulitis is again an emergency. Anti-staphylococcal antibiotics, such as flucloxacillin in combination with penicillin are the recommended treatment.

Theme: Childhood investigations

57. G

Duchenne's muscular dystrophy can be diagnosed by muscle biopsy. The specimen will display the characteristic histological changes.

58. I

Visceral leishmaniasis results in massively enlarged liver and spleen and marrow infiltration. Splenic aspiration to confirm the presence of Donovan bodies is the most commonly used investigation in the developing world, although there is now a tendency to use bone marrow aspiration since it is considered safer.

59. B

SSPE is a late complication of measles (occurring some 10 years after primary infection). It is characterised by an elevated measles specific IgG in the CSF and by characteristic changes on brain biopsy.

60. H

Developmental deficit of ganglions in the myenteric plexus of the colon results in Hirschsprung's disease. The histological diagnosis can be made by rectal biopsy.

Theme: *Multiple trauma*

61. **C**
All this patient's injuries are right-sided, indicating the direction of the impact.

62. **A**
Os calcis and vertebral fractures are typical consequences of a fall from a height. Pelvic fractures may also be caused by this mechanism.

63. **E**
Explosions may cause inhalational/respiratory injuries as well as fractures resulting from the blast. A high index of suspicion is required (continuous pulse oximeter surveillance) with smoke inhalation. The threshold for endo-tracheal intubation should be low as progressive upper airway oedema could make this option impossible at a later stage. Do not forget additional CO and CN poisoning.

64. **D**
This patient has sustained a head injury from striking the windscreen, a fractured sternum from hitting the steering wheel and tibial injuries from dashboard disintegration. He also requires neck immobilisation as he has a cervical spine injury until proven otherwise.

65. **B**
High velocity accidents often result in long bone and pelvic fractures. Motorcyclists are also at severe risk of cervical spine injuries and the helmet should be removed with great care as spinal damage may be aggravated.

Theme: The painful hip in children

66. D

Perthes' disease commonly presents in the 4–9 years age group. It is more common in boys, often with a strong family history. The symptoms tend to be relatively minor in the early stages. At a later stage, X-rays may show flattening of the femoral head caused by localised osteonecrosis.

67. E

This girl has septic arthritis; this condition is characterised by severe pain usually rapid in onset and the child is unable to walk. It occurs most commonly below the age of four years. The commonest organism isolated is *S. aureus*. High inflammatory markers, along with fluid in the hip joint, suggest the diagnosis that is confirmed with joint aspiration. The basis of treatment is surgical drainage with adjuvant antibiotic therapy.

68. F

SUFE is found in older children (boys > girls), up to the age of puberty. Classically symptoms are insidious in onset, as the displacement is gradual. External rotation of the limb at rest is pathognomonic. A special lateral X-ray view will show the posterior displacement of the upper femoral epiphysis.

69. B

Irritable hip often follows an upper respiratory tract infection. The pathophysiology is still unknown. The children develop a form of reactive synovitis in the hip with pain and a sterile effusion. Blood tests are usually normal and the children are not systemically ill. Aspiration of the hip joint will reveal fluid containing white blood cells but no organisms. Aspiration is also therapeutic as it reduces pain.

70. C

Osteomyelitis can be difficult to differentiate clinically from septic arthritis. The pain tends to be more chronic in onset and less severe. In osteomyelitis the child may still be able to walk which is not the case with septic arthritis.

Theme: Cervical disc prolapse

71. **B**
72. **B**
73. **A**
74. **C**
75. **D**

Remember the following landmarks for the upper limb dermatome distribution:

Thumb and radial forearm segment C6
Middle finger (D3) segment C7
Little finger (D5) and ulnar border of hand segment C8
Ulnar forearm segment Th1
Outer upper arm and shoulder segment C5
Inner upper arm and axilla segment Th2 and Th3
The clavicular area (sub- and supraclavicular fossa) is supplied by segments C3 and C4.

Theme: Jaundice in childhood

76. **A**

Jaundice appearing within the first 24 hours of life is nearly always due to haemolytic disease. With the awareness of rhesus incompatibility, ABO incompatibility is now the commonest cause in the UK.

77. **D**

These signs are suggestive of a congenital infection. Congenital toxoplasmosis results in hepatosplenomegaly, thrombocytopaenia, and cerebral calcifications. The children often suffer convulsions.

78. **B**

Biliary atresia is a congenital defect in which there are variable degrees of abnormality of the biliary tract resulting in a progressive obstructive jaundice. Surgical intervention is invariably necessary.

79. **C**

This scenario is very suggestive of breast milk jaundice especially since LFTs and clinical condition are normal.

Theme: Treatment of femoral fractures

80. C

In displaced subcapital fractures the blood supply to the femoral head has been damaged. Fixation of these is therefore likely to fail (avascular necrosis of the femoral head) and should only be considered in young patients accepting the chance that further surgery may be required. In elderly patients the treatment of choice is to replace the femoral head with a hemiarthroplasty.

81. D

Intramedullary nailing is the best treatment as it stabilises the fracture, promotes union and allows early mobilisation and rehabilitation of the patient.

82. B

Below the age of one, gallows traction is very effective.

83. E

In this case the femoral head may be preserved, as the blood supply was probably not interrupted, as there has been no displacement of the fragments. Fixation with cannulated screws should be undertaken within 12 hours of the fracture occurence as the risk of avascular necrosis of the femoral head increases with later surgery.

84. A

These are extra-capsular fractures and the blood supply to the femoral head has therefore not been damaged. Fixation with a screw and plate device such as the Dynamic Hip Screw (DHS) provides much better stability than with screws alone.

Theme: Management of infertility

85. E
86. B
87. C
88. A
89. D

Infertility is a symptom and not a diagnosis. It is often mismanaged with protracted and fragmented investigations. In healthy couples of childbearing age with regular sexual intercourse and without contraception, 80% will achieve a pregnancy after 12 months and 90% after two years. It is therefore not necessary to initiate investigations before one year. Semen analysis is an essential investigation and can be performed in a primary care setting. Two samples one month apart should be investigated. Hystero-salpingogram, laparoscopy and dye test or high contrast ultrasonography will confirm tubal patency.

Theme: Back pain

90. **F**

A sedentary lifestyle is the usual cause of mechanical back pain. The absence of any neurological abnormalities is necessary for the diagnosis. Physiotherapy with back strengthening exercises and postural advice is the mainstay of treatment.

91. **E**

This lady has sciatica. The distribution of her leg symptoms suggests compression of the L5 nerve root which is usually caused by an L4–L5 disc prolapse.

92. **H**

Spinal stenosis causes claudication. The symptoms subside within minutes of sitting down. Assessment of the peripheral circulation is mandatory to exclude any vascular causes. Surgical treatment is by spinal decompression.

93. **B**

This is an emergency. Urgent decompression is required in order to prevent any irreversible damage. The diagnosis is central disc prolapse.

94. **A**

Intractable back pain (i.e. persisting at rest) in an elderly person is unusual. It suggests a malignant process, particularly if associated with systemic symptoms such as weight loss. Spinal tuberculosis is rare in the United Kingdom.

Theme: Short stature in children

95. A

Disproportionately shortened limbs would point to a skeletal dysplasia such as achondroplasia. This is an autosomal dominant condition.

96. G

Noonan's syndrome in boys mimics many of the features of Turner's syndrome however, Turner's can only be found in girls due to the chromosomal abnormality (XO).

NB. XO is the type of chromosomal defect.

97. D

Cranial irradiation especially at a young age can lead to hypopituitarism with loss of growth hormone production and resulting in short stature and hypoglycaemia.

98. B

The child has congenital hypothyroidism.

Theme: Urinary incontinence

99. C
100. A
101. D
102. B
103. E

There are several types of urinary incontinence and the clinical presentation might suggest the correct diagnosis and help to choose appropriate treatment. Urinary fistulae should be suspected after radical surgery or radiotherapy for gynaecological cancers, whereas retention with overflow is common after difficult vaginal delivery (normal or instrumental). Urinary tract infection often presents with urgency and frequency of micturition and must be distinguished from Detrusor instability.

Theme: Chest trauma

104. A

Penetrating injuries to the left lower chest may involve the spleen as this lies under the 9th–11th ribs. Having excluded a pneumothorax on X-ray, this patient requires an abdominal ultrasound to confirm the presence of intra-abdominal bleeding.

105. C

Clinically, this lady has a haemothorax. She is haemodynamically stable and an X-ray is appropriate to confirm the diagnosis.

106. H

This man exhibits the hallmarks of a pericardial tamponade. Cardiac ultrasound will confirm the diagnosis. Needle pericardiocentesis is the required treatment.

107. G

This man is shocked due to a tension pneumothorax. Needle thoracocentesis (second intercostal space in medioclavicular line) will release the pressure and buy time for insertion of a chest drain set.

108. D

This man has a thoracic aortic aneurysm. A computed tomogram followed by angiography will confirm the diagnosis.

Theme: Developmental milestones of children

109. B
110. A
111. D
112. E
113. C

In chronological order most normal children smile at six weeks, sit at six months, cruise around furniture at one year, walk upstairs by two years and are dry by day at approximately three years. All these stages have ranges but in this question there is only one normal age available for each milestone e.g. cruising around furniture is delayed at two years and incredibly precocious at six months so one year is the only possible answer. Major developmental milestones at 6, 12, 18, 24, 36 and 48 months should be learnt for the purposes of the exam. These should be split into gross and fine motor, hearing and speech, social behaviour and play.

Theme: Vaccines

114. E
115. A
116. D
117. C

The UK vaccination schedule should be known for the PLAB exam. The nature of the vaccines is also important for parent information. At present Hib and Meningococcal vaccines are the only conjugate vaccines (a polysaccharide conjugated to a protein carrier) to be used. A simple polysaccharide vaccine in the form of Pneumovax is used for special indications including post splenectomy and immuno-suppressed patients. Measles, mumps and rubella are live attenuated vaccines and although the usual Sabin polio vaccine is a live virus, the killed inactivated Salk vaccine is used for certain patients.

IMMUNISATION SCHEDULE

Vaccine	*Age*
BCG	Neonatal or at 6 weeks
	10-14 years
'Triple' (pertussis, tetanus, diphtheria)	2 months
Repeat **'triple' HiB** and **polio**	3 and 4 months
MMR (measles, mumps, rubella)	12-15 months
Polio, Tetanus Diptheria ('Td') booster	15-18 years
Flu vaccine	65 years (consider yearly)

Theme: Congenital infections in childhood

118. **A**
119. **F**
120. **E**
121. **C**

Congenital infections in children can be very similar in presentation, especially congenital rubella, toxoplasmosis and CMV. They are best differentiated on the basis of eye involvement and the type of calcifications observed. Congenital syphilis results in chronic inflammation of the bones and a bony prominence of the head. Congenital parvoviral infection must be considered in all cases of non-immune hydrops.

Theme: Abnormal smear

122. **B**
123. **C**
124. **E**
125. **D**
126. **A**

The terminology is often confusing. Dysplasia is a histological diagnosis whereas dyskaryosis is a cytological diagnosis. Mild, moderate and severe in both cases equates to CIN I, II and III respectively. A smear during pregnancy and within three months from the end of pregnancy can be misleading and should be avoided unless indicated, e.g. previous severe abnormality. In post-menopausal women and in women who have had a loop biopsy a cytobrush must be used to obtain cells from the squamo-columnar junction.

Theme: Increased susceptibility to infection

127. **D**

In repeated Neisseria infections, complement deficiency, especially deficiency of properdin, a positive regulator of the alternative pathway of complement activation, should be considered.

128. **G**

Opportunistic infections such as PCP are associated with severe T cell defects. All forms of severe combined immunodeficiency have a defect of T cell function and affected individuals are susceptible to PCP.

129. **C**

Although principally conferring susceptibility to bacterial infection, chronic granulomatous disease is also associated with aggressive aspergillus infections and this is one of the main causes of death in this condition.

130. **E**

Although the mechanism is not known, Hyper IgE syndrome (also known as Job's syndrome) is associated with *Staphylococcus aureus* infections. The hallmarks of this condition are severe eczema and high IgE levels.

Theme: Complications of total hip replacement (THR)

131. E

Post-operative swelling in the operated leg is common following THR. Calf tenderness is indicative of deep vein thrombosis. A Doppler U/S scan or a venogram will confirm the diagnosis.

132. D

High inflammatory markers and oozing from a hip wound are hallmarks of a deep infection, such as an abscess. The treatment is aggressive surgical débridement and adjuvant antibiotic therapy in the hope of salvaging the THR.

133. F

Bruising and swelling suggest a haematoma. Occasionally a low-grade pyrexia and mild elevation of the inflammatory markers may accompany these. Treatment is usually non-operative.

134. H

Pulmonary embolism is more likely than chest infection in view of the sudden onset of symptoms. A spiral CT or a VQ scan will confirm the diagnosis.

135. G

Internal rotation, adduction and flexion at the hip are signs of posterior dislocation. This is commonly caused by sitting in low chairs or bending over to pick objects from the floor. In anterior dislocation, the leg is extended and externally rotated at the hip.

Theme: *Skin disease in children*

136. E

This pattern is characteristic of roseola infantum and the rash is exanthema subitum. The causative agent is most commonly HH-V6 (Human Herpes Virus 6) infection.

137. C

Erythema multiforme has a multitude of precipitating factors including bacterial infection (e.g. mycoplasma), viral infections (e.g. HSV infection) and drugs, the most common of which are sulphonamides. The target lesion is characteristic of the condition.

138. B

This is slapped cheek syndrome or erythema infectiosum. It is due to parvovirus B19 infection and is usually a benign condition. In certain cases, especially in individuals with underlying haematological abnormalities it can result in aplastic crises.

139. A

A tick bite from areas inhabited by deer can resulted in Borrelia infection (Lyme disease). The disease progresses in stages but initially leads to the characteristic rash of chronicum migrans. It may progress to meningoencephalitis at this stage.

Theme: Drugs in childhood

140. F

Cefotaxime is now recommended by both the UK and US academic panels as the drug of choice for empirical therapy in bacterial meningitis. Ceftriaxone is an alternative. In younger age groups, amoxicillin should be added to cover against Listeria infection.

141. B

Reye's syndrome is fatty necrosis of the liver that can lead to fulminant liver failure and encephalopathy and is thought to be caused by certain drugs, especially aspirin.

142. G

Cisapride has now been withdrawn form the market due to the concern over arrhythmias especially in association with the –conazole drugs e.g ketoconazole/fluconazole.

143. I

Tetracyclines have long been associated with the staining and malformation of teeth and are not recommended for younger children.

Theme: Genetic defects

144. C

Down's syndrome can be difficult to diagnose in the neonatal period although hypotonia is very common. The presence of duodenal atresia is also very suggestive.

145. H

Short stature and amenorrhoea are the two hallmarks of Turner's syndrome. Both arise from ovarian dysgenesis and can be treated with oestrogen replacement.

146. D

Edward's syndrome (Trisomy 18) is a devastating condition and children usually die in the first months of life. The 'rocker bottom' feet are characteristic of this condition.

147. G

Russell-Silver dwarfism is associated with hemi-hypertrophy and an elfin like face and is the most likely candidate on the list. Noonan's syndrome affects boys.

Theme: Intra-uterine contraceptive device (IUCD)

148. **D**
149. **A**
150. **C**
151. **E**
152. **B**

An intra-uterine contraceptive device is a reliable method of contraception particularly for women in whom oral contraceptives are contraindicated or where there is poor compliance. It should be inserted soon after beginning of the menstrual bleed as the procedure is easier through the slightly soft and dilated cervix and additionally, pre-existing pregnancy is ruled out. Commonest complications are pelvic inflammatory disease, ectopic pregnancy and irregular bleeding.

Theme: Ankle injuries

153. G

This man has a tendon Achilles rupture. The best results in young patients are achieved by open repair of the ruptured tendon. Plaster immobilisation results in weakening of the calf musculature and an increased re-rupture rate.

154. F

Undisplaced fractures of the distal fibula do not require surgical fixation and may be simply treated in plaster.

155. C

Compound fractures require urgent and extensive wound débridement in order to prevent subsequent infection. The use of an external fixator after débridement is preferable to internal fixation techniques because of the lower infection risk.

156. E

Displaced ankle fractures require accurate anatomical reduction if function is to be restored.

157. F

Calcaneal fractures are mostly treated conservatively because of the high risk of wound healing problems and subsequent infections. Only fractures with severe joint involvement are considered for surgical fixation.

Theme: Investigations of postmenopausal bleeding

158. **B**
159. **D**
160. **D**
161. **F**
162. **A**

A gynaecologist should urgently investigate postmenopausal bleeding. Any of the gynaecological malignancies may be the underlying cause. However, they would be unusual symptoms of ovarian cancer.

Theme: Contraception

163. **D**
164. **A**
165. **B**
166. **C**
167. **E**

Most women will go the family planning clinic for contraceptive advice but a proportion will consult their General Practitioner. Progestogen only contraceptives (pill or injection) often cause irregular bleeding but this is minimal. In women with IUCD and a history of pelvic pain and irregular bleeding ectopic pregnancy should always be suspected. Biphasic pills (combined oestrogen and progesterone pill with varying dose of oestrogen through the cycle) may cause breakthrough bleeding and in these cases a normal combined pill should be considered. Rhythm method, i.e. avoiding sexual intercourse during the peri-ovulatory phase has a high failure rate and good compliance requires a high degree of motivation. It is suitable for couples in a stable relationship as failure (i.e. pregnancy) is usually accepted.

Theme: Investigations of pruritus vulvae

168. **C**
169. **D**
170. **A**
171. **E**
172. **B**

In most cases of pruritus vulvae there is an underlying gynaecological cause. However, in a proportion of cases systemic disorders are aetiological factors such as diabetes mellitus or dermatological conditions. Poor hygiene, use of talcum powders, deodorants, bath salts, synthetic underwear, tight jeans and biological washing powders contribute to the symptoms and these should be recognised in the history. In older women with a localised lesion a biopsy is essential.

Theme: Causes of amenorrhoea

173 A

The object of medical treatment of endometriosis is suppression of menstruation e.g. with the contraceptive pill, continuous progesterone therapy or danazol, GnRH etc.

174 C

Premature menopause (i.e. menopause before the age of 45 years) occurs in about 1% of all women; it needs investigating. Possible underlying causes are: genetic factors (family history), chronic infections, metabolic disease (e.g. diabetes mellitus and other endocrine disease), drug treatment (e.g. chemotherapy) or autoimmune disease.

175 B

Amenorrhoea in a teenage girl with normal sexual development but intermittent abdominal pain, palpable lower abdominal swelling and occasionally problems with micturition should make you suspect vaginal atresia or more commonly, imperforate hymen. Colposcopy will show a bulging bluish membrane at the lower end of the vagina.

176 E

Primary amenorrhoea is the correct diagnosis. It has a considerable differential diagnosis, e.g. chromosomal abnormalities (e.g. 45 XO), hormonal disease (e.g. hypothyroidism) and anatomical defects.

177 D

Post pill amenorrhoea is not physiological and if the normal menstruation has not restarted after 2–3 cycles further investigations are necessary. Often the underlying problems are hyperprolactinaemia or other chronic medical disease.

Theme: Vaginal discharge

178. **E**
179. **C**
180. **B**
181. **A**
182. **D**

> History and clinical examination is often sufficient for diagnosis and bacteriological investigations will confirm the diagnosis. Systemic causes and foreign bodies including retained tampons are often the underlying cause. Asymptomatic cervical erosion needs to be treated.

Theme: The painful knee

183. B

The anterior cruciate ligament prevents forward subluxation of the tibia on the femur under normal conditions; its rupture results in instability that is usually associated with a joint effusion.

184. C

Loose bodies most commonly arise in knees of patients with osteochondritis dissecans. In this condition there is necrosis of the subchondral bone with subsequent detachment of a fragment of bone and its overlying cartilage. It most commonly affects the lateral surface of the medial femoral condyle.

185. A

Atraumatic anterior knee pain in a teenager is almost invariably due to chondromalacia. More commonly found in girls who exercise regularly.

186. D

A bucket handle meniscal tear can cause locking (i.e. inability to fully extend the joint). Medial joint pain suggests a medial meniscus problem.

187. E

This is traction osteochondritis of the tibial tuberosity at the insertion of the patellar tendon. It tends to occur in active boys and is characterised by anterior knee pain and tender swelling of the tibial tuberosity.

Theme: Viral infections in childhood

188. B

One has to assume that the child has maternally transmitted HIV and is therefore susceptible to opportunistic infection. Although PCP would be the most common cause, CMV infection can prove equally devastating.

189. E

Post organ transplant patients are immunosuppressed and are especially susceptible to viral infections. This scenario with organomegaly and lymphadenopathy is suggestive of Epstein-Barr related lymphoproliferative disease, which can affect up to 20% of solid organ recipients.

190. G

This child is unlikely to have been immunised and is presenting with an acute mumps infection. Meningoencephalitis represents the most severe complication of mumps infection.

191. F

The umbilicated centre implies that this is molluscum, a benign condition in childhood although lesions may take months to disappear.

Theme: Causes of dementia

192. C

Pseudodementia due to affective disorder may be difficult to distinguish from Alzheimer's disease. In depression the cognitive deficit (if present) is typically acute and recent, whereas that associated with Alzheimer's disease is typically insidious. The depressed patient will often communicate a sense of distress and agitation, and their depression will be associated with other typical features e.g. positive diurnal mood variation and early morning waking. Other clinical features favouring a diagnosis of depression include: family history, previous episodes, and precipitating life events.

193. A

Dementia is a term that describes a progressive and pervasive decline in a number of different cognitive capabilities. A defect in memory is the core deficit in Alzheimer's disease, the commonest form of dementia in this age group. However, individuals with Alzheimer's disease will also show additional impairments either overtly or on examination in other cognitive capabilities e.g. problem solving, word finding and speech, navigation, arithmetic, writing or reading. Alzheimer's disease is caused by a progressive degeneration of neurons in the entorhinal cortex, hippocampus and higher order association cortex, characterized neuropathologically by senile plaques (containing amyloid) and neurofibrillary tangles.

194. F

Post-ictal confusion may produce memory loss, but the onset is acute and associated with symptoms and signs strongly suggestive of an acute seizure.

195. G

Wernicke's encephalopathy represents an acute neuropsychiatric reaction to severe thiamine deficiency. Characteristically patients are globally confused, with gait ataxia and ophthalmoplegia (nystagmus, abducens palsy or conjugate gaze disorder all typical). All three elements of this triad need not be present in order to make the diagnosis. Thiamine deficiency may be secondary to alcoholism, vomiting during pregnancy, dietary insufficiency or gastric carcinoma. Treatment is with urgent intravenous thiamine, but the majority will develop a chronic Korsakoff syndrome.

196. B

Creutzfeldt-Jacob disease is characterized by a rapidly progressive dementia, myoclonus and distinctive electroencephalographic and neuropathologic findings. The infectious agent causing CJD is unique in being a conformationally abnormal prion protein i.e. contains no genetic material. The dementia can be accompanied by signs of involvement of any part of the central nervous system, but myoclonus is particularly common. Although typically occurring sporadically in middle-aged adults, a family history may be present in 8–10%. More recently, variant CJD in young adults has been linked with exposure to beef infected with the bovine spongiform encephalopathy agent. This 'new variant' form often presents with an extended neuropsychiatric prodrome with mood disturbance or other psychiatric symptomatology.

Theme: Drug management of psychiatric disease

197. D

Delirium tremens typically presents acutely after three to four days of abstinence from alcohol. When fully developed the syndrome includes vivid visual hallucinations (not definitely required for the diagnosis), delusions, confusion, agitation and autonomic arousal (often including pyrexia). While short lived (a few days), mortality can be up to 20%. Treatment is fluid replacement and sedation with diazepam or chlordiazepoxide with close monitoring for electrolyte imbalance (especially hypokalemia, but also magnesemia).

198. G

Bipolar disorders consist of a marked change in mood that varies from major depressive episodes to significant manic episode. A manic episode consists of a sustained period (at least a week) when mood was abnormally and persistently elevated, expansive or irritable. Symptoms include inflated self esteem (which may be delusional), decreased need for sleep, talkativeness, flight of ideas, distractibility; they typically cause marked impairment in occupational functioning or relationships with others. The average age of onset of bipolar disorder is about 30 years. Treatment of the acute manic phase is often in hospital. Lithium is not useful in the acute manic of mania, with benzodiazepines (especially lorazepam) being used instead. If the agitation is marked and uncontrolled with medication, it is possible to use ECT to control the manic excitement.

199. A

Symptoms of depression are the commonest psychiatric symptoms in community samples of elderly adults. As with all depressive symptoms, when symptoms become more marked, particularly when disturbing sleep or appetite, then antidepressant medications should be used. In patients who present primarily with insomnia (or agitation), amitriptyline is useful for its sedating effects, particularly given at bedtime.

200. E

Schizophrenia is characterized by psychotic symptoms during the active phase of the illness. Symptoms include bizarre delusions (e.g. involving a phenomenon that the individual's culture would regard as totally implausible e.g. thoughts being broadcast out loud), prominent hallucinations (often a voice commenting on the individual's behaviour or thoughts), incoherent speech, catatonic behaviour and flat or inappropriate affect. During the course of the illness, there is significant deterioration in social functioning and self care. The goal of treatment initially is to decrease symptom occurrence. Medication dosage is increased as long as hallucinations, delusions and disorganized thinking continues; the most frequent limiting factor is the appearance of extrapyramidal side-effects.

APPENDIX 1

In the July 2000 Part 1 exam candidates were provided with a booklet containing normal values for all tests. Below is a short list of normal values as applied to the exam in this book:

Biochemistry

Sodium	135–145 mmol/l
Potassium	3.5–4.8 mmol/l
Urea	2.5–6.7 mmol/l
Creatinine	50–110 µmol/l
Glucose	3.5–5.5 mmol/l
HbA1c	< 7% indicates reasonable glucose control
Bilirubin	3–17 mmol/l
Alanine aminotransferase	5–35 iu/l
Alkaline phosphatase	30–150 iu/l (varies between hospitals)
Calcium (total)	2.12–2.65 mmol/l
Phosphate	0.8–1.45 mmol/l
C-reactive protein	<10 iu/l
Total cholesterol	<5.2 mmol/l (lower if high cardiovascular risk)
Triglyceride (fasting)	<2.3 mmol/l

Arterial blood gases

pH	7.35–7.45
pCO2	4.7–6.0 kPa
pO2	>10.6 kPa
Bicarbonate	24–30 mmol/l
O2 saturation	> 97%

Haematology

Haemoglobin (Hb)	male	13.5–18.0 g/dl
	female	11.5–16.0 g/dl
White cell count (WCC)		4.0–11.0 x 109/ml
Platelets		150–400 x 109/l
Mean corpuscular volume (MCV)		78–96 fl
Mean corpuscular haemoglobin (MCH)		27–32 pg
Red cell count	male	4.5–6.5 x 1012/l
	female	3.9–5.6 x 1012/l
ESR		< 20 mm/hr
HbA2		<3%

APPENDIX 2

A number of drugs are known by different names in the UK to other countries, particularly the USA. Spellings often differ from accepted international spellings. Many of the British Approved Names are to be changed in line with the Recommended International Non-proprietary Names. There are a number of exceptions where the British name or spelling is so well established that either name may be used interchangeably. A few British names have been retained for drugs used in emergency settings, where confusion might be dangerous. In this book, I have mostly used the International name, except for emergency drugs. The lists below are not exhaustive but cover most drugs in common use. A full list may be found in the British National Formulary (BNF).

Drugs where the British name has been retained

British Approved Name	Recommended International Non-proprietary Name
adrenaline	epinephrine
bendrofluazide	bendroflumethiazide
chlorpheniramine	chlorphenamine
frusemide	furosemide
lignocaine	lidocaine
methylene blue	methylthioninium chloride
noradrenaline	norepinephrine

Drugs where the British spelling remains in common usage

British Approved Name	Recommended International Non-proprietary Name
amoxycillin	amoxicillin
beclomethasone	beclometasone
cephalexin	cefalexin
chlormethiazole	chlomethiazole
cholecalciferol	colecalciferol
cholestyramine	colestyramine
corticotrophin	corticotropin
indomethacin	indometacin
phenobarbitone	phenobarbital
sodium cromoglycate	sodium cromoglicate
sulphasalazine	sulfasalazine

APPENDIX 3

HOW TO INTERPRET THE ELECTROCARDIOGRAM

The electrocardiogram should be interpreted in a stepwise fashion. Please make sure that the calibration signal is on the tracing and that it is exactly 1 cm (which equals 1 mV). If the calibration signal is distorted the tracing should be repeated because it can cause artefacts which may be misinterpreted as a pathological change.

Make sure you check the name and, if possible, also the age of the patient.

Modern machines in casualty departments often have a computer programme which analyses the tracings. The programmes occasionally make mistakes, but it is worthwhile reading the interpretation and checking it with your own report.

- **Main axis**
  Normally we only look at the main deflection of the QRS complex. However, it is also important to look at the axis of the P and T-wave which should, with minor variations, be about the same as the QRS complexes.
  The main axis can be easily estimated by looking at leads I, II and III.

  If you find positive (upward) deflections of the QRS complexes in leads I and II the axis is normal. If only lead I has a major positive deflection the condition is called **left anterior hemi-block or left axis deviation**. If the only positive deflection is in lead II and/or III there is **right axis deviation**.

- **Rhythm and rate**
  British electrocardiograms are recorded at a speed of 25 mm per second. A simple way to assess the heart rate is to divide 300 by the number of large squares (5mm squares) between two QRS complexes. We regard rates under 60 and above 100 as abnormal (i.e. the distance between two QRS complexes should not be less than three large squares and not more than five large squares).

  The next thing is to check if the heart rhythm is regular. The commonest abnormality is atrial fibrillation. If there are any doubts about the regularity of the rhythm use a paper strip, mark three complexes and then slide the paper slip along the tracing and compare the distance between other QRS complexes.

Occasionally it is difficult to diagnose atrial fibrillation because there are minor changes of the baseline visible, suggestive of P-waves. P-waves are normally best seen in leads II and VI and if they change their form from beat to beat you are either dealing with an atrial tachycardia or with atrial fibrillation. The distinction between the two states is basically a question of definition and two conditions can show up in the same tracing.

It is important not to miss bradycardia (under 60 beats per minute) or tachycardia (over 100 beats per minute). If you encounter bradycardia you are either dealing with sinus bradycardia or with a conduction defect in the AV node (e.g. 3rd degree heart block).

Please note that 3rd degree heart block often coincides with slow atrial fibrillation and therefore the QRS sequence is irregular. If you encounter tachycardia it is important to distinguish between broad and narrow complex tachycardia. Broad complex tachycardia is usually due to ventricular tachycardia, which is a medical emergency.

- **P wave and P-R interval**
After you have established rate and rhythm assess P-wave and P-R interval. P waves should not be higher than 2.5 mm and should not be wider than 3 mm. If you find wider P-waves you are probably dealing with a so-called 'P-mitrale', which indicates left atrial enlargement due to mitral valve disease. In these circumstances you will commonly find in V1 a bi-phasic P-wave with a prominent negative (downwards) component.

A P-wave which is taller than 2.5 mm is called a 'pulmonary' P-wave or 'P-pulmonale'. It indicates right heart disease with pulmonary hypertension.

A 'saw-tooth' pattern in lead V1 is the hallmark of atrial flutter.

Next, check the P-R interval. P-R interval prolongation of more than one large square is called A-V block first degree. If you have a P-R interval which progressively gets longer followed by an isolated P-wave you are dealing with a Wenckebach block or heart block type 2, Mobitz type 1. If you find a P-wave which is only followed every second, third or fourth time by a QRS complex you are dealing with a heart block type 2, Mobitz type 2.

Wenckebach block is normally regarded as a benign condition. Mobitz type 2 blocks often progress to AV block type 3. In AV block type 3 the P-R interval varies and the patient is profoundly bradycardic (often under 45 beats per minute). The P-waves show no relationship to the QRS complexes.

Remember that slow atrial fibrillation is not uncommon and in these patients you find an extreme bradycardia which is irregular.

In third degree heart block you occasionally also see marked T-wave inversions. If you find very short P-R intervals (< three small squares) you have to consider a pre-excitation syndrome (accessory bundle conduction with intermittent narrow complex tachycardia).

- **QRS complexes**
  For the interpretation of the QRS complex for bundle branch blocks leads I, V1 and V6 are the most important. If you find a widened QRS complex ('sugar cane') in lead I with S-T segment depression you are dealing with a left bundle branch block (often an M shaped QRS complex in V6).

  In right bundle branch block you will find an RSR pattern in lead V1. If the QRS complex is broader than three small squares we talk about complete bundle branch blocks. If it is less than three small squares we talk about incomplete bundle branch blocks.

  Very tall R-waves are found in left ventricular hypertrophy (sum of S-wave in V1 and R-wave in V5 or V6 > 35 mm). If you find a high R-wave in V1 (more than 6 mm) with a deep S-wave in V6 (more than 6 mm) these are signs of right ventricular hypertrophy. An R wave taller than 1.2 cm in AVL also suggests left ventricular hypertrophy.
  NB. You can also get tall R-waves in V1 in the rare isolated posterior myocardial infarction ('true posterior infarction').
  Very small amplitude QRS complexes are found in pericardial effusion, emphysema, obesity and hypothyroidism.

- **S-T segment**
  S-T segment changes are the most important finding in the electrocardiogram. The S-T segment can either be displaced upwards or downwards. Upwards displacement is found in pericarditis, acute myocardial infarction and in an unusual form of angina called Prinz-

Metal angina (coronary artery spasms). Persistent S-T segment elevations (longer than six months) are suggestive of a ventricular cardiac aneurysm or a hypokinetic area.

S-T segment depression is found in myocardial ischaemia, as a digoxin side-effect or in the so-called ventricular 'strain pattern' which is found with right or left ventricular hypertrophy. The S-T segments are also inverted in bundle branch blocks. Remember you cannot diagnose myocardial infarction in the left bundle branch block.

- **T waves**
  Tall, pointed positive T-waves are found in hyperkalaemia, hyper-acute myocardial infarction, occasionally in pericarditis and in young healthy people.

  Negative T waves can be a sign of a sub-endocardial myocardial infarction. They are found in the resolution phase of a myocardial infarction and in ischaemic heart disease without evidence of myocardial death.

  In hypokalaemia little positive waves after the T-waves can occur (U-waves), but occasionally you also find them in healthy people.

- **Abnormalities**
  Q waves

  Poor R-wave progression in chest leads V1–V4 are a sign of previous anterior myocardial infarction.

  S-wave in lead I, Q-wave in lead III and inverted T-wave in lead III suggest pulmonary embolism, but be careful with the diagnosis if the patient is not tachycardic.

  Delta waves in QRS complex are found with a pre-excitation syndrome.

> Always remember: electrocardiographic abnormalities can occur in normal persons without organic heart disease. Organic heart disease, however, may be present in spite of a normal electrocardiogram.

REVISION CHECKLIST

The following themes have recently appeared in the PLAB Part 1 examination. Use this checklist in your revision.

General Medicine
- ❏ Anaemia
- ❏ Antibiotic prophylaxis
- ❏ Causes of acute breathlessness
- ❏ Causes of dysphagia
- ❏ Causes of immobility
- ❏ Causes of pneumonia
- ❏ Chest pain and its management
- ❏ Complications of anti-epileptic drugs
- ❏ Complications of diabetes
- ❏ Decision making in terminal care
- ❏ Diagnosis of acquired liver diseases
- ❏ Diagnosis of asthma
- ❏ Diagnosis of hypertension
- ❏ Diagnosis of infection
- ❏ Diagnosis of joint pain
- ❏ Diagnosis of shock
- ❏ Differential diagnosis of chest pain
- ❏ Haematological diagnosis
- ❏ Headaches
- ❏ HIV risk prevention
- ❏ Hypercalcaemia, treatment and causes
- ❏ Immediate treatment of meningitis/head injury
- ❏ Initial management of convulsions
- ❏ Investigation of chest pain
- ❏ Investigations for headaches
- ❏ Investigations relevant to urinary tract infections
- ❏ Malabsorption
- ❏ Management of arrhythmias
- ❏ Management of breast cancer
- ❏ Management of pain in terminal care
- ❏ Management of stroke/TIA
- ❏ Mechanism of poisoning
- ❏ Method of transmission of infection
- ❏ Pain relief
- ❏ Prescribing drugs in renal failure
- ❏ Prevention of jaundice and hepatitis
- ❏ Prevention and treatment of deep vein thrombosis

- Risk factors of injury in elderly
- Sudden loss of vision
- Swelling of legs
- Treatment of DVT
- Treatment of pancreatitis
- Treatment of pain relief in terminally ill patients
- Unconscious patient

Obstetrics and Gynaecology
- Antenatal screening
- Causes of incontinence
- Causes of vaginal bleeding and primary treatment
- Eclampsia and its management
- Investigations of amenorrhoea
- Investigation for ante-partum haemorrhage
- Investigations for vaginal bleeding during pregnancy
- Management of preeclampsia

Ophthalmology and ENT
- Diagnosis of earache
- Pain in the ear
- Prevention of deterioration of vision
- Sudden loss of vision
- Treatment of earache
- Treatment of red eye

Paediatrics
- Abdominal pain
- Acute vomiting in children
- Asthma
- Bleeding per vaginum
- Causes of vomiting
- Developmental delay
- Difficulty in walking
- Jaundice
- Non-accidental injuries
- Treatment of acute/chronic asthma
- Treatment of urinary tract infection

Psychiatry

- [ ] Acute confusional state
- [ ] Causes of dementia
- [ ] Differential diagnosis of confusion
- [ ] Diagnosis of depression
- [ ] Management of dementia
- [ ] Management of schizophrenia
- [ ] Psychiatric illness and its management
- [ ] Risk of suicide
- [ ] Treatment of alcoholics and drug abuse
- [ ] Treatment of psychosis

Surgery

- [ ] Antibiotic prophylaxis in surgical patients
- [ ] Complications of cholecystectomy
- [ ] Investigations of Acute abdomen
- [ ] Investigations in aortic aneurysm
- [ ] Investigations of a breast lump
- [ ] Investigations of chronic abdominal pain
- [ ] Management of burns
- [ ] Management of an ischaemic limb

INDEX

PASTEST REVISION COURSES FOR
<u>PLAB PART 1</u>

Feeling in need of a helping hand towards success in your exams?

PasTest has over twenty-five years' experience in helping doctors to pass first time, with specially tailored courses to make the most of your valuable revision time.

To give you the most up-to-date information and help you to achieve the best results, we constantly update and improve our courses based on feedback from those who attend.

Our course is run by Consultants and Senior Registrars from leading London teaching hospitals, who have extensive knowledge of their specialty.

Our course material is continually updated to ensure the best possible revision for the exam. You will also receive a complete EMQ mock exam, with explanations and detailed handouts.

- **Course Content**

  Our teaching sessions are based around the PLAB Part 1 examination. The course covers core knowledge, skills and attitudes relating to all exam topics including: Accident and Emergency, Surgery, Medicine, Paediatrics, Obstetrics and Gynaecology, Trauma and Orthopaedics. Our course material includes EMQs with answers and teaching notes, an EMQ examination, tips on examination technique, detailed lecture notes for each subject and a recommended reading list.

Don't just take our word for how good our courses are ...

"Excellent revision course, complete and concise. Top quality lecturers!" Dr Geraldine Sega, Sheffield.
"The course is good, it builds a basic structure on which you can plan all your studies. It really benefitted me – I passed my exam on the first attempt." Dr Ekta Gupta, Solihull.

For queries on books and courses please call our dedicated Customer Services team on **0800 980 9814** or **+44(0)1565 752000**. Alternatively, visit our website at **www.pastest.co.uk**.